the new asylum

a memoir of psychiatry

Frank Prem

Published by Wild Arancini Press

Copyright © 2019 Frank Prem

A version of the poem 'not a lot anymore' first appeared in *Verandah*, Vol 23, (ISSN 1448-4900) Australia 2008.

A catalogue record for this book is available from the National Library of Australia.

Disclaimer: This is a work of creative non-fiction, based on real life events as the author encountered them, through direct experience or observation, or in response to media reportage. Some names, places and identifying details may have been changed to protect privacy and maintain anonymity, and some identifying characteristics and details such as physical properties, occupations and places of residence may have been changed.

Please note that this poetry collection includes occasional coarse language.

There has been no intent to include in this book any cultural or Indigenous references and language, but should any exist, they are included solely for the purpose of telling the story and are not meant to offend, or have any ill intent towards Indigenous culture or people.

Every effort has been made to ensure that this book is free from overt error or omissions. However, the author, publisher, editor or their agents or representatives shall not accept responsibility for any loss or inconvenience caused to a person or organisation relying on this information.

Book cover design and formatting services by Self-publishing Lab

First edition 2019

ISBN 978-0-9751442-8-2 (pbk)
ISBN 978-0-9751442-5-1 (e-bk)

This poetry collection is dedicated to Magdalena and George Prem, who paved the way for me.

I also dedicate it to the patients, consumers, residents, workmates and other individuals who shaped the road thereafter.

Contents

Acknowledgements

My heartfelt thanks to Self-publishing Lab. This is the third collection of my work that has been put together in collaboration with the Lab, and Anthony Puttee, Noel Morado and Penny Springthorpe have been consistently wonderful in their assistance with editing, cover design, contents layout and general advice. I am grateful to each of them for the roles they have played.

Thank you also to my wife Leanne Murphy, for supporting me in these endeavours, always.

prologue

mental-health creature

some things
live within the blood

from when I was a child
riding my bicycle
to visit up top
where my parents toiled
in the old lunatic asylum
discreetly perched
behind the ha-ha wall
I was shaped
to the tasks and functions
of working in mental health

movement into other fields
and naïve dreams
of becoming something
with more glamorous potential
were inevitably fleeting

in the end
after long years
I have come back
and am again that creature
a psychiatric nurse
toiling
in the eternal asylums
of mental health

asylum town

a ha-ha above town

there is always a hill
in a mental asylum town

the ha-ha wall
and the poor fools it protects
and embraces within fine examples
of long-outdated architecture
perches half-concealed
from the gaze
of the good citizens
resident down below

for unlike the near-normal presence
of convicted criminals
in the prison close to the centre
of the township
insanity is unsightly
frightening in the nakedness it reveals
and there is just a possibility
of contagion

atop the hill and behind the wall
out of averted sight
the asylum lies camouflaged
by green acres of gardens
carefully tended
and flourishing farmland
for the production
of vegetables
milk and meat

hidden away despite the prosperity
that a thousand lost souls
living within have ensured
for the past present and future
of the townsfolk
who depend on this location of insanity
to earn
or otherwise access
their daily bread and butter

and it is here
that a young boy's mother
will be shown how to be a ward assistant
and here that his father
will become a kitchenhand in the messroom
and both will learn to be victorian public servants

it is here that the daily journey
to the inside of the ha-ha
above the town
begins

taxi shuttle

every morning
at ten minutes to seven
blue uniforms
starched and stiff
cluster in the spilling light
at the front
of the post office

breath misting
in the pre-dawn cold
of a winter's day

four at a time
in the taxi shuttle
up the hill
for the start
of another shift
in the back wards

first breakfast

for ninety minutes
after coffee
raise them up
out of wet and dirty bedding
then take an allocation
to supervise and assist in the showers
or strip and remake the beds
until breakfast time
for workers and for patients

half staff on first meal break
half on second

then
catch a lift
down the hill to home

thirty minutes
to get the kids up
into the shower
tidy their rooms
and prepare their breakfast
before school

the hoot of a car horn
tells that it's time to go back
to clean the ward again
until first lunch

the smell of stockings

there is a particular odour
that attaches itself to feet
when the shoes are removed
at the end of a thirteen-hour day
which begins
with the tepid sloshing waters
of showers and baths
for forty-five incontinents

the leather of nursing shoes
captures moisture
and holds it
in a tight-fitting soup
that surrounds feet and winter hose
as the day goes on
with cleaning and washing floors
in the clammy warmth
of a steam-heated ward

my mother wants only
to take off her shoes
to rest swollen
and painful feet

I
want to leave
the room

conditions of employment

conditions of employment
say a man can't make extra arrangements
with any other employers

it has to be
one day rostered on
one day rostered off
in the heat of the main kitchen
and that's all

but at the end of a summer
when the weeks of hot sun
have done their work
and the crops
have reached a ripening

when pollen and storm warnings
are filling the air

there's a farmer in porepunkah
with thirty acres of grass
to cut for hay
and to cart into storage
before the rain spoils it

and in the stanley hills
there are orchards
with their own brief seasons
of apples and pears
and sweet black cherries

to be picked and graded
and packed for cool storage

while the plumber
in town
needs an able assistant
to dig ditches
erect spouting
and perform general handiwork

there's a house to pay off
a refrigerator to buy
and the kids are wearing mud
into the neighbours' carpets
because there is
no television at home

conditions of employment
don't understand
the conditions of living
that a man with a family
has to meet

sunday lunch on the ladies ward

oh hello dear
how are you
don't you look lovely

I'm not sure if I look lovely
but they sound strange
like little girls boxed up
inside old ladies

it's sunday
and I've jumped on my bike
and gasped my way
up to where mum is working
in one of the female wards

the women always seem
to be kept busy there
scrubbing or mopping
or folding something
but they're all over me
when I visit

almost petting me

mum is really pleased
when I ride up
but sort of hurries me away
out of the main room
like she's not sure it's good thing
for me to be there

in an empty dormitory
I perch on a neat bed
feet swinging
while mum ducks out for a second
then comes back
with a plate of roasted chicken
left over from lunch

and pink junket
for a special sunday dessert

spreading magic

dad is in the bread room today

out of all the places I've been to
the bread room
is the best

he pops me up on top
of a couple of huge boxes of butter

more butter
than anywhere else in the world

then he loads up the machine

a loaf of white sandwich bread
is placed for slicing
and the softened butter
set for spreading

the machine starts up
and as the bread gets sliced ...

... it comes out buttered

oh boy
no hands

magic

Frank Prem

a hundred dollars every week

long days of work
on aching legs
and run right off her feet

home at last
to yet another round
of wash and clean

never a spare smile
to lighten
a femininely handsome face
and no moment
for a breath of peace

always something
one more something
yet to do

day after day
long into the evening
no change
to the way it is

except for a teardrop
that forms in her eye
when the little boy
with a small voice asks

mama
when I grow up
if I can earn
a hundred dollars a week
do you think my wife
can stay at home
and not have to work every day

card collector

there are many ways
to collect a set of cards

medals of war
types of poultry
butterflies
or flags
from countries
all around the world

it can be as slow
as eating five vita brits
almost more than I can hold
every morning

that'll get me two cards
every couple of weeks
with good health
and extra-vitamin strength
as a by-the-way

it can be faster
when my mum's right there
to open the packets
for breakfast on the ward

six cards in a single day
makes the smile
of a hot collector

but a better way
that has to be the best of all
is to talk to old eugene
the man who has control
of the most cards
in the whole wide world

when I ride up
to the hospital store
and ask him
he waves me right inside
points me to the ladder
and I can open new packets
until five o'clock

two hundred cards
in my pocket
and I'm the best
there ever was

student daze

would you consider ...

I'm sorry
we don't have any vacancies
for cleaning staff

but
we're about to commission
a new acute psychiatry unit

would you consider
being a student nurse

a student psychiatric nurse

wearing the colours

cooks must be gleaming white
ward assistants dull blue

nursing sisters are fawn
while their aides
shine brightly
in lime

it's loam brown
for the gardeners
and the overalls
of engineering are navy

girl student nurses are pale sky
while male nurses
like me
are drabs
in their nondescript grey

for a long time

we huddle in a group
while the secure door
is unlocked to admit us

a small man
with wild grey hair
and unmatched eyes
wearing a rumpled shirt
greets us
sing-song style

hello boys and girls
how are you all today
are you visiting the wards
on your first morning
that's lovely

who is he

what did he do to get locked up

he looks so strange
has he been here long

that
oh prospective students
is the nurse in charge
of the locked ward

he has been in charge
for a

very

long

time

the most important thing

a final-year student
is acting as our guide
to the units that comprise
this institution

between mental-retardation wards
known as children's cottages
and psycho-geriatric wards
he instructs
on the critical knowledge
we will need
to survive our training
and to care
for our patients

you have to remember

he says

to wipe
away from the vagina
when you're cleaning up
a female patient

otherwise
you might cause an infection

what

WHAT

pecking order

each table holds ten
eight tables allow eighty
at each sitting

on the far side
is the matron's table

matron at the head
then the senior female nurses
arranged around her
with junior nurses
seated down the sides

none to commence eating
until matron does

in the centre
are the artisan staff

engineers
tradies
domestics

men and women
each to their segregated tables

on the near side
male nursing staff sit
as per their pecking order

my student group
are the current fools
of the institution

we sit anywhere
boys and girls together
oblivious
to stern
disciplinary glances

character formation

we are the student intake
to be formed into
modern
psychiatric nurses

to be taught
with the new psychology

in week one
we are rolling on the floor
bodily over each other
stating loudly
quack
quack
as each colleague
passes across

in week two
we are urged
to open our souls
and bare our secrets
to one another
in intimate
team-building exercises

in week three we are told
there has been a mistake
your group contains
one student
too many

the group must decide
which one of you
has to leave

in week four
we are commencing
an abiding association
with alcohol

token economy

first-year students
are not allowed
much responsibility

but I am in control
of the ward cigarettes

a cigarette after a shower
a cigarette to behave
a cigarette for helping with the cleaning
a cigarette for singing a song

my life is taken over
surrounded
by the cigarettes and smoke
that make this world
go around

while I
poor fool
decided to stop smoking
just a week ago

Frank Prem

where the air

when it rains out there
we smoke
in here

thirty of us

gradually
the dayroom fills
smoke descending from the ceiling

until the only air available
is gasped
by lying full length
on the floor

but still
we smoke

to pharmacy for tubes

the deputy-in-charge
has sent me on an errand
to pharmacy

the morning clinic
cannot proceed
without a specialised item
of medical equipment

ask the pharmacist
he instructed
for a pair
of fallopian tubes

the pharmacist laughs
says I should ask
one of my female colleagues
for a loan

Frank Prem

a dead parrot

the old and enfeebled
are seated
in a quadrangle of chairs
placed in the centre of the dayroom

aged schizophrenics
and dementias

*... this is a dead
parrot ...*

disembodied discussion
about a prone norwegian blue
fills the ward
from end to end
through overhead speakers

today's in-charge
is a monty python fan

the rest of us
better learn to be

toilet routine

twenty minutes to lunch

time to toilet the psycho-geriatrics

some are wheeled to the bathroom
then transferred to a commode

some are helped
into a cubicle

one mumbles to herself

mum mum mum mum
mum mum mum mum

and leaves wet sock prints
all the way from her lounge chair
down the corridor
and into the bathroom

for her
the signal that it is toilet time
is also the signal
to wee

cleaning up

charlie is a veteran
of two train crashes
and a spot
of incidental brain damage

a tiny bit
foul-mouthed

sister schmidt
is a charge nurse
german
a disciplinarian

the linen is stacked
according to straight lines
and tight rules
in sister schmidt's ward

charlie
is having a word
you're a fucking old blurgl urgl

sister schmidt
with flannel and soap in hand
is washing his mouth

no language like that
in sister schmidt's ward
thank you
very
much

famous flying choppers

it is after dinner
six o'clock
in the oldies' ward

my colleague
carries a tray
holding fifteen silver cups

each cup contains
a set
of pearly whites

uppers
lowers
uppers and lowers

students
collect the teeth
after each meal
and scrub them
in the laundry sink

but the tray
when placed too close
to the edge
is unstable

and
not for the last time
in student history
the choppers fly

sleeping

it's night duty
the ward is sleeping

male patients
in the men's dormitory

female patients
in the women's dormitory

staff
on chairs in the lounge
on the sofa
in the staffroom

I walk the corridors
watch patients squirming
in fresh-piddled beds
that cannot be changed
until the ward round takes place
near dawn

it's night duty
the ward is sleeping

birdies at mealtime

two of us
supervise the mealtime queue

a woman
talking back to voices
preoccupied and distant
reaches across
takes my colleague's hair
in one hand
and drives her head
into the solid wall

the woman collects a meal
wanders to her chair
and commences eating
still preoccupied
with inner voices

my colleague
is trying to follow the path
of a flight of colourful birds
circling her head

Frank Prem

bathing the locked ward

twenty-five hunched
pigeon-chested little men
run naked
across the cobbled winter courtyard

to the bathroom
dip
dip
dip
in and out
of the peninsula bath

one is faecal
for him
the shower
and a stiff scrubbing brush
on a four-foot-long
extended handle
to prevent splashback
onto the nurse

the room is steam
and smell

row your boat

a tall gaunt man
from the retardation wards
wanders the grounds daily

nondescript overalls
and absent socks

in a world of his own

I see him spread
a white table napkin
on the ground
take a seat on it
and begin to rock
as though rowing a boat

he leaves the napkin behind
when he wanders away

drawn in blue ink
to fit the boundaries of his canvas
are the boards
seat and oarlocks
of a rowboat

a day at the races

the ward outing
is at a local racetrack

patients onboard
staff onboard
food supplies onboard
alcohol onboard

the quantity of beer
is heroic

all drink freely
a good time is had

the return trip
is an hour of smells
incontinence
and vomit

some of it
is even due
to the patients

getting stuffed

a man has died

I am learning
that it is nurses' work
to prepare the body

I understand
sponging down

and ticketing a label
to a toe

I can make sense
of the slack body

the difference
that absence of life
imposes

and I realise the point
of inserting wadding
into loosened orifices

but
I cannot comprehend
the rage
of the senior nurse
as she manipulates
the gauze with tongs

and there are no explanations
in my texts
to account for her need
to apply such a vicious
final insertion

in charge of retardation

the room is all women
dumpy and thick
short and spherical

dilantin gums
oversized and swollen
holding no teeth

me with thirty women

the moment the evening meal
is finished
all thirty of them
are disrobing

their clothes flung
through the dining-room window
to the ground outside

I am surrounded
by a wriggling
grotesque
fleshy tableau

and no conception
of what I am meant to do next

or where
I should look

medication jam

medication time
in the retardation ward

there is a line
four metres long
of joyful anticipatory faces
queued up
like traffic delayed
in peak hour

one at a time
they shuffle forward
to receive a large dollop of jam
with tablets enclosed

placed deliberately
onto each tongue

and wiped clean
by sticky lips

bounce and flow

a manic young woman

she is in seclusion
jumping up and down
up and down
in front of the window

to hold my attention
she has taken off her top
breasts
going up and down
up and down

she moves around the window
making sure
she keeps me focused
on her actions
up and down
up and down

later
when the water seeps
under the wall
destroying the carpet
I realise
she had stuffed towels
and tissue paper
into plugholes and toilet pans
then let the water flow
and flood

while she bounced
for me

up and down
up and down

huntington's marionette

she is young
perhaps forty years old
but in with the psycho-geriatrics

huntington's chorea
makes her dance
in a long slow death
that steals the mind
before it takes the body

she is drooling
incontinent
disgusting

and for the duration
of a six-week-long
rostered placement
has possession
of my breaking heart

better than that

wanda is middle-aged
close-eyed
and manic

her mouth is going
ninety to the minute

she can't stop
can't rest
can't leave anything alone

babble babble
fiddle fiddle

SLAP!

she has hit me
open-handed
across my face

there is a grin
hiding just in the corner
of those glittering eyes

and I want to
strike her down

but as a good nurse
I remind myself

for weeks
I remind myself
that I am
that I have to be
much better
than that

Frank Prem

after the ball

the annual asylum ball
is a dying tradition

this could be the last
so we have drunk and eaten
danced and fallen
talked nonsense
through a long night

one nurse
has popped out of her dress
while performing a vigorous
two-step

her dance partner tried
unsuccessfully
to help return all offending items
to their intended locations

but his wife didn't approve
and took him home
early

now
here I am starting work
at seven in the morning
and have not gone home
have not changed clothes
have not slept

leila who is in charge
of the medical ward
has seen it all before

takes me in hand
and lays me down
for a few hours kip
in a vacant bed

come back
she says
when you're awake
and sober

after asylum

final discharge

in its serenity
the town cemetery is a beautiful place
the granite work and the statuary
hold a sombre dignity
in the peaceful air

a contrast
to unmarked mounds that are
little more than gentle blemishes
in the waving grass
that surrounds a wandering path

many histories lie here
pioneer spirit and gold
plague disease and chinese ceremonial
anglican
jewish
catholic
and unwanted

on the left side
towards the back
inconspicuous and out of the way
are those unclaimed who are
at last
in possession of their final discharge

released
from the paternal care
of the mental asylum

consumers now

in the game
they're referred to
as consumers now
with service delivered
to a place called home

but I used to know them
a little better than that

they were
ella and ferdie and max
and eddie and pinky and b-ee-ill

they're long gone
and never come to mind
except on visits
to deserted dayrooms
and haunted dormitories

managing: acute observations

opening the door; surveying the realm

this is not a locked ward
it is classified
open: acute
I checked

but I am standing
waiting
for staff to open up
and let me enter

to notice that I am here

there is a gaggle of them
talking in the nurses' station
too busy
to pay attention

~

and this is it
my new ward
the ward of rumour
and innuendo

the place of raised eyebrows
and a muttered
good luck
when it is mentioned
when my new role
is spoken of

this is that place

so many lost souls
directionless
falling under the sway
and barely existing
within these crazy walls
day after day

it seems tragic

and then
there are the patients

a doctor for the seclusion room

why you have me here
why is six men around me
I am not skizofrenia
in my country I am doktor
you understand
woman doktor

jravay ko krednost prjavno

no I not speaking you english
no no
leave me
no
ayiiiieee do not injection
why you attacking me

zloa zloa ariboch slao
ao ao

ayiiiieee
I am doktor
I am not sick
let me go

zloa zloa zloa

let me home

the weed of rights

he said

that's not really a joint
you know
it's just a kind of
tobacco
with green

and I know it's not the usual shape for a
roll-roll-roll-your-own cigarilla
but it takes all kinds
and if I want to use up my cigarette papers
that way
I think that's my business

~

he said

well alright but
I didn't smoke it

you caught me too soon
and I only would have taken a puff

what harm
can a single puff do to you or me
we are men of the world
and I've smoked this stuff
daily for thirty-two years

so have you
I bet
haven't you

come on you can tell me
my friend

we are both men

~

he said

it was only for me
just a private device for my mental health
I don't know
how that other guy got any but
I'm no dealer
I'm not
look at me look at me do I look
like a dealer

no
I'm an honest man
honest like the sun in the sky
the length of a day
you can trust me
my friend

I would never do that

~

he said

but that's bullshit
you know there's no truth in that tale
I'm not ill
I am well
and the doctors those bastards
have no business to be holding me here
against my will
I could sue them you know
and I might just do that I will sue them
for having no right to hold me
to treat me with pills and injections
while denying these things
that I need

I want my release
want my freedom
want out of here and you
please
give me back my weed

oh
you're all bastards and shits
go away
I thought I could trust you but
you're a bad man
as bad
just as bad
as the rest

you are not good

not a lot anymore

we're standing in the staff courtyard
it's break time
and we're doing coffee and a cigarette
when he says to me

I've always worked in psych
I love it

I've never been tempted
by anything else

it's changed though
from the old days
oh
a hell of a lot really

he takes a deep drag
lets out the blue smoke
of a reflective moment
has another sip
from the styrofoam cup
and says

you know what

about a year ago
we had a real old-fashioned case come in
like we used to get
in the old days

no drugs
no family history
no obvious causes
just crazy

mad as a cut snake actually

it was a first presentation
and it took a while
but we fixed him up
he got better and we turned him loose
he hasn't been back

that's what I like best
good straightforward madness
that you can do something with

but you don't see much of that
anymore

shook up; looking better

she's looking better
seems to know now
how to make a smile appear

I think she's getting better

we first met in her room
on a visual-observation round
two weeks ago

she held a flashlight
with a long string tied to the end
looked guilty
confessed that the string
was a fascination
she was trying to release

perhaps she could run it round her neck
pull tight

pull tight
then slip away

but I think
she's looking better now

~

she's been fasted for anaesthesia
her pills withheld

walks slowly along the corridor beside me
not speaking

up on the trolley
a name band
no jewellery
no false teeth
no nail varnish

into the theatre suite
to sleep

relax the muscles
monitor heart check breath
dab the goo onto the electrodes

go

a shudder
some twitches

go

on to recovery

recovery

~

she's still quiet
had a late breakfast and the morning meds

looks a little shook up
but I think
she's better

yes
I think she's a little better now

kickstarting the morning

it was over before it started

I'd never seen this guy before
not to say hello to
not to medicate
not to upset

no interactions

and I wasn't close to him
three or four feet away
not even looking at him

but he said hello
in his own special way

my colleague told me it was nothing
and she was right

she said it's just how
he announces himself
and I could see
that was true too

she said he'd never intended
to make contact
and I had to agree
he'd missed me
after all

but she couldn't quite convince me
that the kick he straightened out
just above my shoulder
an inch or two from my jaw
before turning around and walking off
was the right way to say
good morning

act-ed up

you get sentenced
to thirty days
maybe forty

the act can do that to you

one day
you're walking the streets
minding your business
listening to your voices
running amok a bit in a quiet way maybe
or just sitting alone in your room
for a few weeks
a month

doing no harm

next thing
someone makes a request
and some doctor you've never seen before
seconds the motion with a recommendation

[SNAP] you've been section 9'd
and the police cart you off to the inpatient unit
in the back of a divvy van

[SNAP] you've been section 10'd

some psychiatrist confirms involuntary status and
[SNAP] you've been section 12'd

to get force-fed pills
injections
not allowed to leave
hardly to breathe or scream
until a doctor says it's okay
okay

OKAY

IT'S NOT OKAY

NOTHING
is
OKAY

there's a guy here
only twenty-two
he's already done a hundred days
and he'll do a hundred more
god help him

that's your act for you
your bastard mental health act

ah
you're all nothing but a pack
of pricks

the eyebrows I think

it made for an almost feminine appearance
in a strictly masculine face

as though he'd applied heavy makeup

but it was actually just the eyebrows

funny how you don't notice them at first
just the look of a stranger
on someone who is actually familiar

disconcerting

he'd done half his head as well
hard to know where the obligations begin and end
with someone who is a patient
held against his will

fashion policeman
doesn't come within the standard
nursing job description

I told him the female staff
and some of the patients
were complaining about him
masturbating all over the place

I said he should keep it in his pants
and to act like an adult
or he'd end up in seclusion

he asked
but what about when my pants slip
and I have to grab them
showing me with one hand on the waistband
and one cupping his jewels

or
what about if I'm walking
and just need to ...
scratching in the general vicinity

nope
I'd have none of it
I told him

he looked vaguely disappointed
tried out another
what if ...
before focusing on a cigarette
and mumbling about not meaning to ...

I never quite got
what he wasn't meaning to ...
I'm a little deaf
and he's a little brain damaged
and it was just a passing discussion
distracted by the absence
of eyebrows

black visitor

the black cat lies
in the doorway of the unit
she doesn't seem
to be after treatment

and I don't believe she's come to call
on anyone residing
behind the doors

this is the summer season
and the sun beats down
on the bricks and on the mortar
baking the concrete that surrounds the unit
and encloses us

the shouting is contained
but I can decipher every word I hear
as he screams out loud
to the bursting of his lungs

you bitch

he cries

you whore

he sends a wish for
suicide
that reverberates around the walls

Frank Prem

do you like it

bitch whore

you kill babies

this is the summer season
and today there's a black cat
lying on her back full stretch

enjoying warmth
under a golden sun

she looks happy
but then
I don't suppose
she's after treatment

I don't suppose
there's anyone she wants to see
and I wonder
who could blame her
for that

duck chocolate and tapas

we're opening
with tapas
but I don't know what tapas is

in a faux-spanish restaurant
there are eight of us
a small gathering
drawing breath
in the middle of a crowded week

and it begins with a platter
of marinated ribs
some sort of fried calamari rings
cheese and special-sauce potatoes

olives

they call it tapas

~

a mother
out near seymour
on the edge of the catchment
is staring at her meal

the food tonight
came out of the freezer
but it wasn't touched
by either of them

it's been pushed now
towards the centre
of the dining-room table

she's still dressed in her better clothes
hasn't changed
it was a long trip to the hospital
and she's too weary to bother

the boy
her young man
was a mess today
still so ...

sick
strange

frightening

she thinks
thank god
he's in the inpatient unit
but
what are they doing for him

he isn't getting any better

what can they do

this is the worst
it's ever been

what's going to happen

she cries silently
and knows even as she weeps
that she's the strongest of them
it will destroy her husband

she is the stronger
and she is weeping

wishes they hadn't visited
perhaps it will be better
tomorrow

~

the deep red
is a delicious warmth
and the conversation flows

a joke about the service

a word about the practice of medicine

thoughtful comment
on the demography of the area
how we differ
from the adjoining catchments
rural versus metropolitan

familiar faces pass by
to settle at neighbouring tables
and there's comfort to be found
a sense of belonging in this place
on this evening

our rural city seems
undisturbed by the fall of night

the waiter has removed the tapas
platter empty
and now
we're waiting for the mains

it's all very pleasant

the last olive was mine

~

things are jumping
on the unit

it's full up
no beds
but there's another patient
with an overdose
a psychosis
drug related
anorexic
old

something

it doesn't really matter what
there's always another one
and tonight there'll be an argument about it
the night shift aren't happy with the triage team
and they make a stand

if you want to leave another patient with us
you better find extra staff
because we haven't got enough
and we won't do it

I don't care who says so
we've got too much to do
keeping that young yahoo you just brought in
under control

if there's no extra staff
there's no going over numbers

okay
welcome aboard for the night shift

don't worry
the manager can sort it out
tomorrow

our job is to keep that crazy bugger
under some sort of control

~

chocolate duck is an unusual dish
rich and rewarding

our table is silent now
almost

there's only the clinking of cutlery
an occasional appreciation

and the sound of an ambulance
disappearing into the distance

idle thoughts
idle thoughts
I always stray back to the job

the petty worries I can do nothing about
but can't help overworking

the main dishwasher
in the unit's kitchen
has broken down
what will it do to the budget
if I replace it

is there a choice
nope

perhaps I should raise the salary level
of the new nurse
she's working out well enough

they'll be shortstaffed in the morning
the roster's deficient
I hope someone's put their hand up
to fill in for the absentees

I wonder if the sickies are real
or just bludging

might need some help with that one

fingers crossed the boy from seymour
doesn't cause too much grief
he'll be a bugger till we can get the drugs
out of his system

his drugs out
our drugs in

oh well

it's all pointless
I can't do anything until tomorrow
and talk at our table is starting up again

this has been a nice way
to end the day
duck
chocolate

tapas and all
I still don't know
what tapas means but
I might get to work it out
tomorrow

h.r.t. fan

a staff nurse mentioned today
in passing
it's been sixteen years
since they took out my
ovaries and uterus
and all that

it was just a conversation
about a fan she'd misplaced
and how she needs it every day
every hour sometimes
when the flushes rise

she woke in the middle of the night
last week
to find herself
saturated
pillow sheets and nightwear

the doctors have told her
that's the way it has to be
unless she restarts hormones

but she doesn't want that
they don't feel safe to take
and she's had lumps removed already

she knows a friend
a woman
who's been having flushes

for over thirty years
and probably will forever

if anything
is forever

meanwhile
she wants her fan
now
and if one of the male staff
has hidden it
there'll be hell to pay

phew
sometimes
it gets pretty hot around here

lost: one cockerel

he's a skinny little kid
is this one

wiry
you'd call him

every so often
he lets out a scream

bloodcurdling really

the first time
you want to race down
to the seclusion room
and check to see that he's alright
never mind
if it's time for the fifteen-minute obs
or not

but he just smiles
a big whole-of-face
and all-of-teeth smile
says no
it was just the devil he was yelling at
he's fine really

o ...

... kay

~

the little bugger has turned the bed upside down
it's a solid block of foam rubber
on its arse in the corner of the room now

sheets and blankets are everywhere
but at least he's peed into the bottle
and hasn't gotten into any
fingerpainting

last time that happened
an aboriginal guy rendered
the national coat of arms
kangaroo and emu and shield
all over the wall in shit

it was that good
I almost saluted

~

four hours is up
time for the mandatory medical exam

lord he's a dag
grinning at us hugely
with his eyes full of trust
and a complete absence of guile
but utterly unpredictable

when the doctor wants to put her stethoscope
onto his chest for a listen
he puffs himself up like a little cockerel

~

we've been through anti-psychotics
nothing has worked

we're doing shock therapy
but he's already too high

we've kept him away from illicit substances
he's not using

we've nursed him in high-dependency
and in seclusion
to keep stimulation low

no effect

he's not much more than a kid
this bloke
but I think his life is shot to bits

we've lost him
already

frankly no worries

some of the patients
the young men mostly
call me franky

it's a mixture of familiarity
and respect
because they know I'm the manager
the boss
with a separate office
and different work

they know
I don't dress
the way most of the staff do
often tell me
I look more like a doctor

but they know
too
that they can talk to me
chew my ear if they want
that I'll try to find them a spare moment
out of my day

it's a funny job
hard man one minute
uncompromising while I lay down the law
state what I will and won't tolerate
outline the consequences
hide any doubts I might feel

then next moment
I'm telling a joke
laughing
showing that I have an idea or two
about where they're at
and why they want to rampage
over their anger and frustration
their distress

they can call me franky if they want
I guess
I can live with that

no worries

this somebody's boy

and he talks to me
this young man
in a babble of words

I say nothing
he's too high

a touch of macho
surrounding an elevated mood
racing fast and furied
until he stops

suddenly

dead quiet

and his face starts to move
into creases and crinkles
reshaping while he struggles
his eyes go glassy

and then it's all sadness
this boy
this somebody's little boy
is doing it tough

because it's hard to be a man
all the time

a well-honed team

ah no
no no no
this is all over the place

I don't believe what I'm seeing
what I'm involved in

there are ways to do this
simple ways
six staff
two for arms
two for legs
one for meds
and one talker

only one talker

but we're all over the place
there are three staff talking
arms and legs have been left behind
and have to push past all the talkers
if they're going to perform any kind of restraint

the patient is in a corner of the room
bed on one side
wall on the other
so we can't get near her

and whoever went to fetch the injection
has been gone an age

this is supposed to be slick
to minimise distress
minimise risk

what the hell is going on

trained professionals
that's us

ha

ha

ha

that's all (last saturday)

jesus doesn't live in bed north eight

he might have visited on saturday
that's all

that's all

the room is empty but for a bed

but for a blanket

but for the pillow
of a lonely girl
who believes something
she can't explain
except to know
it isn't jesus anymore

no

he might have been a visitor last saturday
but that's all

the carer meeting

they are mainly older people

making tea
getting the biscuits
familiar with one another
from months or years of meetings
like lions club
or rotary

one or two
look a little startled
half afraid

new to the game

~

I am meeting with a group of carers
have been asked to seek their views
about service provision
and they are ready to tell me
have rehearsed and repeated their stories
many many times

no longer expect to get a response
but are happy to speak anyway

being listened to is cathartic
even if nothing happens

the stages of a career in caring
for the mentally ill
are transparently on show

~

the newbies look stunned
haven't come to terms with what it means
this intrusion of mental illness
into previously unsuspecting lives
not yet comprehending the future that awaits them
only wanting to know
what is wrong
how to fix it
and that help will be there for them

does anyone know what this is
this schizophrenia
why has it happened
why now
did we do something wrong

will it happen again

~

the middle stagers are angry
but to say that doesn't do them justice
ropeable is better
they know they won't get service
when they need it
that no beds are available
unless a life is at stake

that you have to be half beaten up
or expecting to die
before anyone gives a shit

the only way to get a response
the only way mind you
is to park your car
in front of the ambulance entrance
at the emergency department
and not shift it

if you want to get them to do anything for you
you have to inconvenience them

they're supposed to be professionals
to help those who need them
but they just don't care

not until it's too late

~

the old hands have seen it all

they're angry too
but
they've gotten to know the system
over the years

understand that the staff do their best
some better than others
but generally they do what they can
to make it work

when you've been around
twenty or thirty years
as some of us have
you learn things

like that you'll be managing
and untangling
this bloody sickness for the rest of your life
the rest of your loved one's life anyway
so you better adjust to that

you learn where to put your finger
to get at the pulse of influence
the senior doctor
the executive officer
the local member of parliament
you keep at them to change
but you plan it out
brace yourself for the long haul

you have to make sure you keep enough strength
to manage your own ups and downs
look after the newbies
hose down the others
and keep the pressure on

be sure they don't add any policies
or make stupid changes
they haven't asked you about first

we rely on each other in the group
to keep going

but never mind that
would you like a cup of tea
before we start

so young man
what is it that you
want to ask us about

and the hell with the papers

yes
and in an illusion of sanity
I made piles of paper
out of piles of paper

I picked up stack after stack
flicked through them
as quickly as I dared
to determine which had the potential
to bite me
which were likely to be benign

separated those
that were personal

and I threw them
bundle by bedraggled bundle
behind the swivel
on which
my working world turns

let them rot there for a day
a week
until I tire
of their un-filed clutter

safe in the knowledge
that there is no prospect
of lingering importance
in their yellowing ink lines

it isn't a great system
I know
but this is the first time
the first day
in many months
that I have seen the green inlay of my desk

and it makes me grin
with foolish pleasure

I don't care
what I've not yet responded to
nor whom I may be causing to wait
or to have to rewrite a request

this
has been
for me

what happened

she said
look
I wasn't planning to throw a sickie
halfway through the day

what happened is
I was going home for lunch
and I saw my son
I told you yesterday
about him having that chronic thing
that might turn out to be cancer in his gut

the poor little bugger is only seventeen

anyway I saw him sitting on the fence
around the corner from home
and he was howling his eyes out

he's tried so hard to be brave
but he just couldn't hold it in
so I gave work up for the day
I'm sorry
that had to be my priority

I knew he was pretty sick
but I've tried to sort of protect him
from the facts of it
until I was sure just how bad it was
and could explain it all to him
but that fucking surgical registrar

excuse my language
but oh they're such clever doctors
and absolute fools as people

he just blurted it out
as though he was talking to an adult

there's a hell of a difference
between seventeen years and fifty
when you're being informed
you might have a cancer

I'd be grateful if you'd tell the other shift leaders
that I might need time off at short notice

if I speak to them myself
I'll just start crying again
and that wouldn't be any help to anyone

I don't know what's going to happen

I'll let you know

from long black shoelaces

I think they're going to pull the plug soon

maybe tomorrow

she's been in intensive care since thursday
in the afternoon
when we found her
tried to bring her back to life

she started breathing by herself
for a while
but that's all

today they said her brain has died
everything is being done
by machine

set to automatic

on friday
we talked amongst ourselves
spoke about what we thought had happened
what we saw

someone said it looked too late
before we'd even started

and the nurse who cut her down
had already lived this
once

this was her second one
the same all over again

why do they do that

I don't know
nobody seems able to say
but this girl used shoelaces
lost consciousness
then strangled

it seems a stupid empty way to go
and today
we've been remembering
that suicide is a fleeting thought
and our job
is to see folk through
to the other side of
nothing left
worth living for

a community-based colleague
said she was thinking of us
as she drove to a home visit
when
halfway around a bend
she saw a mother cow
licking a baby calf

and around the next
a flock of cockatoos
the biggest she's ever seen

and she thought of us
checking bedrooms and bathrooms
for people suspended
maybe dying
thought she was lucky in her work

I guess she is

tonight
I got a call from intensive care
family members want the possessions
the diary and phone numbers

I'll carry it all across the campus
tomorrow morning

but the shoelaces
have gone

between ridiculous

it's a fine line

we're saving a woman
from killing herself because
her life
is a form of dying

she says if she has to go on
it's not worth it
she might as well pull out the picc line
that delivers liquid nutrients
to feed her
and just bleed for a couple of minutes
till it's over

a very fine line

sometimes it makes sense
to be thinking in terms of
an ending
I can understand that
yes I can

no really
I can

when life is reduced
to never tasting food in your mouth again
never being allowed
to bounce a grandchild on your knees

lest you start bleeding
and always always having the bloody picc
to remind you that you're an invalid
yes
I can understand

and the anger too
to have your life destroyed like this
through simple mishap
during a routine procedure
in the operating theatre

I know about the anger

it's just that
before you can decide
it's not worth it
and that you want
to pull the plug
you have to be sane

and if you're miserable
because your life seems to be
in a terminal state
of appalling
that's not sane
it's a depression we have to treat
before you can do
what you have to do

you can't be allowed to kill yourself
unless you're of sound mind

the line doesn't get any finer

~

the medication
and the shock therapy
have shaken her memory to the foundations
she's started writing little notes
just to try to catch up
to the place where she was
before treatment

her husband helps
reminding her of what has gone before

and she may not have improved

but
how can we choose any better
between what's rational
and what's mad
even when I think
that I too would rather die
if I were in the same position

I can't imagine
never being able to eat real food again
or living the whole of the rest of my life
through an intravenous drip

and in the meantime
the treatment has to go on

I wish she and her husband
would remember that
and not hold us responsible
for shooting her memory
into such very small pieces

or blame us
for not letting them act
on understandings they've reached
about what to do
when it becomes intolerable
it's no good pointing the finger
we're only trying to help her
to be rational
when deciding

it's a terribly subtle line
really

~

one of the nurses told me
that there's been a murder
a double suicide
up in the hills
the details were in the local paper

in the end
sometimes
sanity prevails

raising the pride

today they're okay
on this day at the start of october
I'm proud

this crew of mine
a random ragtag of workers
has pulled together
to make it through the shift

it wasn't without drama
sickness left our numbers down
experience was light on the ground
and there was madness in the air

hallucinated voices insinuating

hooch smoked out of sight of everyone

trouble brewing behind brooding looks

and a young guy rocking non-stop

he's out the back
in the high dependency
with a head full of trouble
so wrecked
that we don't know what to do
and maybe there's nothing we can do

I'm not sure what will become of him

but today the shift held up
they worked for each other
for the people they're here for
and it went okay

I feel proud

nursing theory

well alright
if you really want to know
I'll tell you the theory
my theory

see
a few eons ago
they stopped making people like me

I'm a relic from another time

I rubbed shoulders
with madness and eccentricity and violence
and plain nuttiness
for three full years before they licensed me
to be a psychiatric nurse

nowadays
if they give students two or three weeks
it's a luxury

back then
they figured that
if we could treat really sick people
in their homes or in the community
those people wouldn't need to come to hospital
the treatment could go to them

fair enough

so what happened
was that all the nurses who had a few runs
on the board
skills and experience
went off to work in the community

well you would
wouldn't you

lovely

except that the result
and you don't need to be a rocket scientist
for this bit
the result
is that we started getting the sickest people
the ones
that couldn't be managed in the community
coming into the inpatient units

drug-induced psychosis
violent
resistive
suicidal
homicidal
bloody near impossible

at the same time
we stopped training people
in the way they'd created nurses like me

oops

no wonder it's a bloody struggle
for the poor buggers working in the acute units

no wonder it's hard to find staff

you can't blame them for not being interested
in learning on the job in psychiatry

and no wonder the system is stuffed

anyway
I don't know if there's a place in the game
anymore
for an old fart like me

I'm too cynical
jaded maybe
but that's my theory
some other bugger might tell you different
but one thing's sure

it isn't right

weary

and I give them so much of myself
everything I can
until my head is a spin
of issues and events
of decisions and repairs
plans and predictions
treatment and containment

I give them all I have

and it is not enough

never quite enough

I am
so
tired

meandering journey

this one's a story
about travelling
and never really knowing where
until arrival

only to find
that it's time again
to keep moving on
in a restless way
that's littered with small
shining gems of meaning
waiting to be stumbled upon
if your eyes stay fixed
firmly on the ground

pick a day

pick any shining day
you like
you might choose the one
we just had
why not
it was bright
and the sun rose

there was a woman in my ward this morning
I had to tell her
that she was welcome
but that there really wasn't much
I could do

her ills and ails
were beyond my reach and ken
but I would do all that I knew how

she smiled

it took away her pain
for the moment
that we shared
and my impotence
was a thing
we could both laugh about

the light of truth
was more palatable
than the darkness
of yesterday

sometimes I think
the only thing there is
that keeps us hanging on
and clinging
to a shining thread
is the laughter
that emerges from the night
when we speak honestly

I'm sorry
I've meandered
but this is still
a travelling poem
and I am moving
to another place

today it's true
I stopped a while
but it was temporary

hostel life

the hostel princess sings of her future with eric the nurse

strum-strum-strum-strum
strum-strum-strum

eric nurse loves me
eric nurse loves me
he's going to take me away
we'll live in a castle

I am a princess

strum-strum-strum-strum
strum-strum-strum

eric nurse loves me
eric nurse loves me
he's taking me
to my castle

I love to live
in my castle

I am a princess

strum-strum-strum

the other one

paul
paul
I'm sorry I yelled at you before paul
but it wasn't me
it was the third one
inside my belly

it was the other one paul
it wasn't me

she always calls me paul
gets easily confused
among the various male nurses

moments ago
she was screaming at me
a berating sprinkled with suitably dire threats
and heartfelt curses
because I'd refused to make yet another cup
of coffee

a tempest
whipped up and blown out
in a few banshee breaths
then the regrets

I'm sorry paul
you know it was that other one
in the middle

she points a finger to her abdomen

I'm only six years old paul
I shouldn't have to take
all these tablets

she tucks back an unruly mass
of stringy grey-streaked hair
fixes her gaze
somewhere beyond my left shoulder
and wanders outside
in search of another cigarette

mad till knock-off

they're mad today

~

al·len is calling me *fran·kay*
over and over
because he likes the sound of it

fran·kay ha·ha·ha

fran·kay ha·ha·ha

~

get in the shower bob

use the soap bob

wash under your arms bob

wash between your legs bob

wash your behind bob

use shampoo on your hair bob

bob will be leaving soon
moving on to independent living

~

lisa has stolen some money from staff
and they're talking about it around her
as though she's not present

looks like her paranoia is rising
says one

it's obvious
she's agitated because she's feeling guilty

if we just keep on for a while
she'll give it back
she won't hold out for long
when she knows
that we know

~

the little gnome
is having an ultrasound on an ulcer

in the car he bops
like a teenage fiend

he absorbs the music
of saturday morning video shows
and now the radio
has tuned him in

go-go little gnome
just you go

~

paul
paul

she still calls me paul

I didn't take it
the other one took it

be nice to me paul

paul
can I have a cold coffee
and my cigarette

please paul

~

they're all mad today

hurry up
knock-off-work o'clock

Frank Prem

furball and freddie

furball the tabby
is a calamity
of sorts

add up his losses and you get
just about half
of one cat

the tail is gone
an ear
the eye on the left
is quite blind

but he's been a part
of the institution for years
and every so often
one of the staff
gets him trimmed up
and shaved

until he becomes a slender peculiarity
that merges at the front
with an oversized fluffy head
like an egyptian sphinx

quite alarming to the uninitiated

furball's day
is in and out of the houses
and stalking birds

generally smaller
than the black-and-white ibises
that reside in the backyard

it's not a bad life
when all's said and done

~

freddie was romanian once
way back when

migrated his aspirations
to the mental asylum
of a very small town
in australia
and grew old there
before he came to us
in the hostel

sometimes he cries aloud
inconsolable like a baby
in torn-up romanian
or maybe he's not even using
the words he was born with
just voicing an anguish
only he feels

in the bedroom
his personal touch
is the skeleton
of a piano accordion

the bellows are ghosts
and the buttons have sagged
deep into the frame
leaving just the holes
as suggestions

but it's there and it's his
perhaps it brings to mind the memory
of some far-distant polka

da-dat-da da-dat-da da-dat-da
da-da-daddle-da-dat-da

except for what's inside his head
he's a complete loner
and I couldn't guess
what might be happening in there

~

tonight
on the medication round
I surprised him
already in bed
and I couldn't help noticing
that freddie does not
sleep alone

before rising to face me
he tucked in and settled furball
the cat with no ear
with no eye
lacking tail

medicine gulped
the two snuggled up with a purr
in romanian
as I turned out the light

I'm sure it was meant as
goodnight

cigarette? still laughing!

she's a stroller
with teeth
falsies that shine bright
like ill-fitting pickets
behind a rictus of lips

and that particular laugh
heh heh Heh HEh HEH
HEHHHH!!!
that would work best
around a cauldron
in a group of three

with thunder

beady-eyed chief scrounger
her stroll is always
in pursuit
of an unfinished cigarette
a butt end that can be manipulated
to provide the elusive last drag
or a light
to get the
puff-puff
damn thing going

on sunny days
the cackle
filters down the slope of the yard

from where she reclines
on the hostel's broken chaise lounge
and chortles to a private amusement
at the apex position
that commands a view
of every likely location
and repository
for a careless discard

retrieved swiftly
like a bright flash
of descended lightning
while the fag end still bravely salutes
with the rise of a sinuous blue wisp

oh yes
this is the good life

heh Heh HEH
HEHHHH!!!

the tweedle man

they dress him in braces
that hold his jeans up
to just under his chest

with a red cap on top
he is baby brother
to the tweedles
both dum and dee

specially built boots for club feet
adjust a walking slant
that can't make up its mind
to be either a jaunt
or a topple in progress

under the cap is the devil of a grin
and the gleam from his eyes
could be a boy's glass marbles
peeping out from a close-held bag

but

ohhhh
look at my pants nurse

it's an outrage
to be wet again

ohhhh
look nursey

look at my pants

who's going to change him

ohhhh

and after that
the notion is unspoken
but shared between us
that it's ever so much better
dear nursey
sweet nurse
much much better
to be dry

he slant-saunters away
hidden somewhere under the brim
of his hat
tweedle-ee tweedle-ay
tweedle-um

before breakfast

these four are a hormone

then
there's one for your blood
a small one so you piddle
two to get you sorted
down below
and in behind

the purples are for mood swings
the green one my dear
is just because you're mad

and in case of a side effect
well
here's another one

hold out your hand
it's like a fist full of lollies
isn't it

there's gob-stoppers
all-sorts
jellybeans and smarties
plus
a drink with some fizz

be careful
don't fart

no don't ask
just swallow them down
dear

I'll get you a slice of warm toast
with marmalade

enjoy your breakfast

under the skin

they are morphogenetic twins
with only superficial differences
disguises to mislead the inattentive

cardigan overlay
streaky grey hair
stare-over-the-shoulder eyeballs
    dumpy
    platinum-blonde wig
    wide and thick
    red lipstick

instant VOICE PROJECTION
    instant VOICE PROJECTION

piercing **SHRIEK**
    piercing **SHRIEK**

it's not my fault paul
it was the other one that did it paul
I'm only six years old
    It's not my fault frank
    it was bella inside me she did it
    I'm only twenty-three

can I have a smoke
it's time for my smoke now paul
    frank will you get my smoke now
    I want my smoke now frank

oh you're such a BASTARD paul
get out get out GET AWAY FROM ME
I HATE you
>   *I am SO going to marry robert*
>   *he DID NOT write that he wants me out of his life*
>   *I HATE you frank you're a BASTARD*

hahahaha I like you paul
you're not too bad
>   *I really like you frank*
>   *you're nicer than those other nurses*

good night paul
>   *good night frank*

yes
goodnight my dear girls
sweet dreams

cracked-pepper clinic

fra-ank
she says it with a sing-song inflection at the end

fra-ank
an insistent entry
into my consciousness

I'm driving back from the nearest city
where we have attended the fracture clinic
two weeks ago she fell down some stairs
and received a tiny crack in one toe

the receptionist beckoned to me
after registration
do you know what she told me her name was
she said it was autumn
autumn summer

we agreed that autumn summer
would be quite a nice name at that
and smiled knowingly at each other

now here
on the drive back to the hostel
she has been watching me closely for twenty kilometres

fra-ank

   ye-es

when we get back
can you do something
on your computer

    what is it you want me to do

could you fix up the pepper in my head

oh

    what does the pepper inside your head do

you know
she says
it goes round and round
and stops me from reading and from writing
will you get on the computer and fix it

    well of course I will
    as soon as we get back
    to the hostel

looking forward to a homecoming

yes
I can tell you what happened

yesterday
she took off her clothes
and started walking around
in the corridors
and past all the other residents
again

the senior nurse noticed
and asked me
to do something about it
so I took her by the hand
and led her to her room

she even smiled at me a little
though there's not much expression
on her face

well
we entered the room
and oh
she was as quick as quick
and without any warning
she turned her hands over
and dug her nails into my wrist

really hard

I screamed
the pain was excruciating
and she forced me down to my knees
by digging harder

I thought she'd cut
right through
to an artery

it took all three of the other nurses
that I was on duty with
to prise her fingers out of me

oh
I was a hell of a mess afterwards
don't worry about that
blood and tears
emotional trauma

gob-smacked

all last night I was nearly hysterical
and my husband got so angry
I think because he felt helpless
swore he wouldn't let me go back
to work

the thing that stuck in my mind
was the way she stayed silent
showed nothing on her face
and yet I could tell she really meant it
really meant to hurt me

yes
I'm at work again today
I mean these people need care
don't they
and someone has to do it

but enough of that
how is she going in the acute unit
when is she likely to be discharged

we need to get ready
for when she comes back home

parfait crazy

I'm sitting with a mental illness
she could be schizophrenia
she could be
manic d
bi-polar
a druggie full of voices in her head

but right now
she's a parfait glass of chocolate
topped with cream
and dripping syrup

I'm a flat white

so I'm sitting with an insanity
and refreshments
at a pavement table
wondering what to say
but I know there's nothing
except
are you ready to go back yet
and I know she is

I've been sitting with a mental illness
she's a crazy
I've no doubt it's true
but it seems that I'm the one
who's paying

praying m

fra-ank
fra-ank

she comes my way
the peroxide-blonde bombshell
who is all red lipstick
ghost foundation
and a tottering
half-moccasin shuffle

last heard screaming

you're a bastard
you're nothing but
a bloody fucking bastard

in the context of my failure
to adequately distribute her ration
of cheap menthol gaspers
every hour
on the hour

fra-ank
can you help me frank
I've got a praying mantis in my hair

well
that one
is a conversation stopper

and sure enough
there clings
a fourteen-centimetre-long
bronzed-copper beastie
looking well at home
in the outlandish
fine but brittle
coif

they like me
they do

they look at me
all the time
in the smoking shed

they stare
but they like me

happy chronicity

and we're a car full of chronics
on the way to a clinic
to see an authorised doctor
and get the clozapine renewed

beside me
she's babbling in a balkan conversation
that needs no other speakers
but a fellow traveller in the back of the car
is solicitous

are you alright
rosie dear

another guy with a german name
is pushing me beyond distraction
with a fiendish prattle that features
some interaction between cows
and scottish bagpipes

billy-boy completes the number
they're playing in my head
through applied philosophy
when he asks the question

frank

are you happy

epilogue

still its creature

in aftermath
it seems so clear

there are few mental-health
happy endings

and there are no
simple cures

there's just the risk
of cynicism
among repeat offenders
with bad habits

and minds that won't
take the time
to learn

there's only so much
before enough
of trying to change worlds

enough of listening
catching flak
and shouldering tears

of bearing
other people's burdens

there is no room
no role
for heroes

this is only mental health
and all it requires is you
and I
to be its creatures

Psychiatric Support and Counselling

If reading the material in this poetry collection has caused emotional distress, or if you believe that you or anyone you know might need help, in Victoria (Australia) contact one of the following support services:

Service	Focus	Phone number	Operating hours
Emergency	Emergency assistance	000	24 hours/7 days
NURSE-ON-CALL	Expert health advice from a nurse	1300 60 60 24	
Area mental health services triage	Generally the first point of contact for people seeking a specialist mental health response that will identify the urgency and nature of response required	Phone numbers are available in each area	24 hours/7 days
Beyond Blue	Depression, anxiety and related disorders	1300 22 4636	24 hours/7 days
Lifeline	Crisis support, suicide prevention and mental health support services	13 11 14	24 hours/7 days
Mind Health Connect	Directory of mental health support and resources	N/A	24 hours/7 days
SANE	People affected by mental illness	1800 187 263	9–5 weekdays
ARAFEMI Carer Helpline	People affected by mental illness	1300 550 265	9–5 weekdays

If you live in another Australian state or territory, or another country, search for *'mental health counselling and support services'* online to find help in your area.

About the Author

Frank Prem has been a storytelling poet for forty-five years. He has been a psychiatric nurse through all of his professional career, which now also exceeds forty years.

He has been published in magazines, online zines and anthologies in Australia, and in a number of other countries, and has both performed and recorded his work as 'spoken word'.

He lives with his wife in the beautiful township of Beechworth in northeast Victoria, Australia.

If you would like to read more about Frank and his psychiatric experience, additional articles and background can be found on his website: www.FrankPrem.com.

Newsletter

Subscribe to Franks newsletter to receive news about forthcoming publications and writing activities, also at www.FrankPrem.com.

Other Works by Frank Prem

Small Town Kid (2018)

What readers have said about *Small Town Kid*:

A modern-day minstrel. Highly recommended.
—A. F. (Australia)

Small Town Kid is a wonderful collection. Cover to cover, this is an excellent read.
—S. T. (Australia)

Frank's style is minimalist, with plenty of room to fill in the blanks with your own conjecture or possible parallel memories.

Written about an Australian town that was a gold-rush town in its day, it touches on those times as well as describes the landscapes there. Frank's work is approachable, understandable, and sensitive in its handling of the most delicate of subjects.
—J. L. (USA)

Devil in the Wind (2019)

What readers have said about *Devil in the Wind*:

Trust me, this book will stay with you. Bravo!
—K. K. (USA)

Very moving, beautiful, and terrible. I was left with a profound sense of respect, as well as a reminder that we should never take for granted every precious every moment of life.
—J. S. (South Africa)

Outstanding! Beautifully written, the author has given a human voice to those who matter. Highly recommended.
—B. T. (Australia)

CPSIA information can be obtained
at www.ICGtesting.com
Printed in the USA
BVHW040833141019
561030BV00013B/102/P